MW00509233

THE
COMPLETE
LOW-CALORIE
COOKBOOK

Table of Contents

As promised, please use your link below to claim your 3 FREE Cookbooks on Health, Fitness & Dieting Instantly

https://bit.ly/2MZF09w

You can also share your link with your friends and families whom you think that can benefit from the cookbooks or you can forward them the link as a gift!

© Copyright 2018 by Charlie Mason - All rights reserved.

The following Book is reproduced below with the goal of providing information that is as accurate and as reliable as possible. Regardless, purchasing this Book can be seen as consent to the fact that both the publisher and the author of this book are in no way experts on the topics discussed within, and that any recommendations or suggestions made herein are for entertainment purposes only. Professionals should be consulted as needed before undertaking any of the action endorsed herein.

This declaration is deemed fair and valid by both the American Bar Association and the Committee of Publishers Association and is legally binding throughout the United States.

Furthermore, the transmission, duplication or reproduction of any of the following work, including precise information, will be considered an illegal act, irrespective whether it is done electronically or in print. The legality extends to creating a secondary or tertiary copy of the work or a recorded copy and is only allowed with express written consent of the Publisher. All additional rights are reserved.

The information in the following pages is broadly considered to be a truthful and accurate account of facts, and as such any inattention, use or misuse of the information in question by the reader will render any resulting actions solely under their purview. There are no scenarios in which the publisher or the original author of this work can be in any fashion deemed liable for any hardship or damages that may befall them after undertaking information described herein.

Additionally, the information found on the following pages is intended for informational purposes only and should thus be considered, universal. As befitting its nature, the information presented is without assurance regarding its continued validity or interim quality. Trademarks that mentioned are done without written consent and can in no way be considered an endorsement from the trademark holder.

INTRODUCTION

I want to thank you for purchasing *The Complete Low-Calorie Cookbook.*

In a world that is easily lead of-course to better health by temptation and a lack of self-discipline, it's difficult to stay on track when it comes to fueling your body like the temple it is.

We all wish we were healthier, whether it be we had more muscle, looked leaner, weighed less, exercised more, etc. The unfortunate thing is, many of us never find the motivation required to get on the path to becoming the best version of yourself, both inside and out. We become stuck in a rut of unhealthy habits that many never remove themselves from.

If you are ready to make a change to your life, this book filled with delicious, low-calorie eats is exactly what you need to start your journey living a healthier life.

While there are hundreds of books that showcase delectable low-calorie meals and treats, this one is short, sweet, and to the point. It was created with efficiency in mind. All dishes included are less than 300 calories per serving and take less than an hour to make. We focused on providing you with recipes that withhold optimum ingredients and have easy-to-follow directions.

Thanks again for choosing this one! Every effort was made to ensure it is full of as much useful information as possible, please enjoy!

BREAKFAST RECIPES

1. Muffin Tin Eggs

Calories 172 – 9g Fat – 1.8g Carb – 21g Protein

Servings: 6

Ingredients:

- ¼ tsp. marjoram
- ¼ tsp. red pepper flakes
- ½ tsp. pepper
- ½ tsp. salt
- ½ tsp. sage
- ½ pound fat-free ground turkey
- 1 tsp. steak seasoning blend
- 1 diced bell pepper (red, orange, or green)
- 12 eggs

Instructions:

1. Ensure your oven is preheated to 350 degrees. With non-stick spray, liberally spray a muffin tin.

2. Spray a skillet and add ground turkey. Mix in marjoram, red pepper flakes, salt, pepper, and sage. Cook 7 to 10 minutes till cooked well.

3. While turkey mixture cooks, beat eggs and steak seasoning together 2 to 3 minutes till fluffy. Stir in diced pepper.

4. Spoon cooked turkey mixture into greased muffin tin. Pour egg mixture over turkey mixture, filling eat compartment ¾ full.

5. Bake half an hour.

2. Pumpkin Spice Smoothie

Calories 112 – 7g Fat – 2g Carb – 11g Protein

Servings: 2

Ingredients:

- 1 tsp. pure maple syrup
- ½ tsp. pumpkin pie spice
- 2-3 dates
- 1 C. unsweetened vanilla almond milk
- 1 banana
- ½ C. pumpkin puree

Instructions:

1. Split banana into pieces and add to a blender. Add all remaining ingredients.
2. Blend mixture till smooth in texture.
3. Taste and add additional sweetener as needed.
4. Serve sprinkled with a pinch of cinnamon. Enjoy!

3. Honey Almond Energy Bites

Calories 90 – 8g Fat – 0.5g Carb – 16g Protein

Servings: 10-15

Ingredients:

- 1 C. oats
- ¼ C. peanut butter
- ¼ C. honey
- ¼ C. chopped almonds
- 1 tbsp. flax seeds

Instructions:

1. Spray a mixing bowl with cooking spray. Add all ingredients to mixing bowl and combine well.
2. Roll mixture into small balls. Place on baking sheet and into the fridge till you are ready to eat them.

4. Sweet Potato Breakfast Bowl

Calories 190 – 11g Fat – 5g Carb – 12g Protein

Servings: 1

Ingredients:

- 1 tsp. cinnamon
- 1 ripe banana
- 3 tbsp. almond butter
- 2 tbsp. almond milk
- 1 large sweet potato
- Extra virgin olive oil

Optional Topping:

- Fresh blueberries
- Cinnamon
- Almond milk

Instructions:

1. Wash potato and pat dry. Peel and slice in half lengthwise.
2. Ensure your oven is preheated to 400 degrees.
3. Drizzle potato slices with olive oil and place them on a baking tray and into the oven.
4. Bake 30 minutes till soft. Remove from oven.
5. Toss sweet potato into a food processor. Add a dash of salt and remaining ingredients. Blend until thick but soft.
6. Pour into a bowl and heat in microwave till warm. Transfer to a serving dish and add desired toppings.

5. Raspberry Apple Granola Bars

Calories 167 – 7g Fat – 3g Carb – 13g Protein

Servings: 12-18

Ingredients:

- 5/8 C. diced unsweetened frozen raspberries
- ½ C. unsweetened applesauce
- 1 C. rolled oats
- 1 tsp. melted coconut oil
- 1 tsp. cinnamon
- 1 tbsp. honey
- 5 tbsp. skim milk

Instructions:

1. Ensure your oven is preheated to 350 degrees. With cooking spray, spray a baking pan.
2. Mix applesauce and coconut oil together till smooth. Then mix in honey, cinnamon, and milk till thoroughly incorporated.
3. Stir in oats and then raspberries.
4. Pour mixture into prepared pan and press down gently.
5. Bake 16 to 19 minutes. Allow to cool to room temperature before enjoying.

6. Easy Breakfast Burrito

Calories 257 – 10g Fat – 6g Carb – 17g Protein

Servings: 6

Ingredients:

- ¼ tsp. cumin
- ¼ tsp. chili powder
- ½ C. reduced fat shredded Mexican cheese
- 1/3 C. enchilada sauce
- 3 sweet potatoes
- 15-ounce can black beans
- 1 avocado
- 8 egg whites
- 6 low- carb whole wheat tortillas
- Red pepper flakes

Instructions:

1. Wash and dry sweet potatoes. Pierce with a fork. Place in microwave and heat 4 to 6 minutes till soft and cooked through. Set to the side to cool and then place into a bowl. Mash with forks till soft.
2. Drain black beans and rinse with water. Let dry.
3. Place black beans in a bowl and add cumin, chili powder, and a few dashes of red pepper flakes. Stir till well incorporated.
4. Cut avocados lengthwise. Separate meat from skin and slice into cubes.

5. Add egg whites to another bowl, beating well.

6. Spray skillet and add egg whites. Cook and fold on occasion to strive for a fluffy texture. Remove egg whites from heat when cooked.

7. Warm up tortillas with the same skillet.

8. While tortillas are warm, divide sweet potatoes between them and spread. Do the same with black beans, shredded cheese, and avocado.

9. Drizzle with enchilada sauce and season with pepper and salt.

10. Roll up tortillas. With parchment paper, line a tray and place burritos on it.

11. Bake 5 to 10 minutes.

12. Serve with sour cream, Greek yogurt, salsa, and/or hot sauce.

7. Pumpkin Pancakes

Calories 151 – 3g Fat – 2g Carb – 7g Protein

Servings: 8-10

Ingredients:

- ☒ 1 ½ tsp. apple cider vinegar
- ☒ 1 ½ tsp. vanilla
- ☒ 2 tbsp. coconut oil
- ☒ 3 tbsp. pure maple syrup
- ☒ 2 eggs
- ☒ ¾ C. pumpkin puree
- ☒ 1 C. unsweetened almond milk
- ☒ ¼ tsp. Nutmeg
- ☒ ½ tsp. cinnamon
- ☒ ½ tsp. salt
- ☒ 1 tsp. baking soda
- ☒ 1 tsp. baking powder
- ☒ ¾ C. coconut flour

Instructions:

1. Combine all dry ingredients. Then add all wet ingredients and incorporate thoroughly with a hand mixer.
2. Spray a pan with cooking spray.
3. Spoon 2 tablespoons of batter into pan and cook 3 to 5 minutes per side till browned.
4. Continue process with remaining batter.

5. Serve pancakes with maple syrup, a dollop of butter and a dash of cinnamon.

8. Tropical Orange Smoothie

Calories 79 – 0.5g Fat – 2g Carb – 3g Protein

Servings: 1

Ingredients:

- ½ C. almond milk
- ½ C. frozen pineapple
- 1 banana
- 1 orange

Instructions:

1. Place all ingredients into a blender and blend on high 60 seconds till smooth.

9. Banana Berry Smoothie Bowl

Calories 143 – 5g Fat – 8g Carb – 9g Protein

Servings: 2

Ingredients:

- ½ C. unsweetened almond milk
- 1 C. spinach
- 1 C. mixed berries
- 1 banana

Optional Toppings:

- Berries
- Banana slices
- Toasted coconut
- Almonds
- Chia seeds
- Coconut granules

Instructions:

1. Peel and cut the banana into slices. Place into the freezer overnight. Do the same with mixed berries.
2. Wash and dry spinach. Cut into small chunks.
3. Add frozen banana and berries to a blender, adding almond milk and spinach. Blend until a smooth texture is created.
4. Add mixture to a bowl and top with desired toppings.

10. Raspberry Zinger Energy Balls

Calories 167 – 7g Fat – 3g Carb – 13g Protein

Servings: *16*

Ingredients*:*

- ☒ 1 C. shredded coconut
- ☒ ½ C. almonds
- ☒ ½ C. raspberries
- ☒ ¼ C. almond butter
- ☒ ¼ C. dried cranberries
- ☒ 4 dates

Instructions*:*

1. Add ½ a cup of coconut to blender and pulse till it turns to a crumbly mixture. Set to the side.

2. Add remaining coconut to a blender along with remaining ingredients. Process on high till combined.

3. With parchment paper, line a baking tray.

4. Take a tablespoon of raspberry mixture and shape each into balls. Coat each ball in coconut crumbs, ensuring all sides get coated.

5. Place coconut coated balls on a tray and chill 2 hours.

LUNCH RECIPES

1. Honey Mustard Chicken with Bacon

Calories 298 – 5g Fat – 20g Carb – 25g Protein

Servings: 5

Ingredients:

- 2 tbsp. chopped parsley
- 1 tsp. cornstarch
- 1 C. skim milk
- 1/3 C. light cream
- ½ C. cooked/diced bacon
- 1 tbsp. olive oil
- 1 ½ tbsp. minced garlic
- 3 tbsp. whole grain mustard
- 1/3 C. honey

Instructions:

1. Mix a pinch of salt, oil, garlic, mustard, and honey together. Coat chicken in honey mustard mixture.

2. Fry bacon and then sear chicken in the same skillet till eat side is just browned.

3. Add remaining mustard to the pan as chicken cooks with cream and milk. Heat mixture to simmer till chicken is completely cooked.

4. Remove chicken and mix cornstarch with a tablespoon of water and add to pan, mixing till the sauce becomes thickened.

5. Place chicken back in skillet and coat with sauce.

6. Serve topped with bacon and parsley.

2. Turkey and Bacon Lettuce Wraps

Calories 102 – 4g Fat – 8g Carb – 10g Protein

Servings: 2

Ingredients:

- 1 thinly sliced Roma tomato
- 1 thinly sliced avocado
- 4 slices cooked bacon
- 4 sliced deli turkey
- 1 head of iceberg lettuce

Basil Mayo:

- 1 chopped garlic clove
- 1 tsp. lemon juice
- 6 torn basil leaves
- ½ C. gluten-free mayo

Instructions:

1. To make basil mayo, mix together all mayo ingredients in a food processor till smooth.

2. Lay out your lettuce leaves. Layer 1 slice of turkey and spoon on basil mayo. Then layer a second piece of turkey with bacon and a few slices of tomato and avocado.

3. Season a bit with pepper and salt then fold the bottom up and roll. Cut in half and serve cold.

3. Chicken Bites

Calories 295 – 15g Fat – 7g Carb – 21g Protein

Servings: 5

Ingredients:

- ¼ tsp. pepper
- ¼ tsp. salt
- 1 tsp. garlic salt
- 1 ½ tsp. paprika
- 1 C. coconut flour
- ¼ C. cream
- 3 eggs
- 1 ½ pounds boneless, skinless chicken

Instructions:

1. Cut chicken into slices.
2. Combine cream and eggs together.
3. Add chicken slices to cream mixture and set aside.
4. Add pepper, salt, garlic salt, paprika, and flour to a plate. Combine with a fork.
5. Dip each chicken piece into the flour mixture and add to heated skillet with coconut oil.
6. Cook chicken 3 minutes and flip. Place on plate with a towel to get rid of oil.
7. Sprinkle with additional salt and devour.

4. Chicken Salad Pita

Calories 300 – 9g Fat – 12g Carb – 19g Protein

Servings: 1

Ingredients:

- ☒ 1 whole wheat pita
- ☒ ½ C. chopped chicken breast
- ☒ ½ grated apple of choice
- ☒ 1 tsp. low-fat Greek yogurt

Instructions:

1. Mix together yogurt, chicken breast pieces, and apple till combined.
2. Stuff whole wheat pita with chicken mixture.

5. Garden Pasta Salad

Calories 299 – 11g Fat – 15g Carb – 6g Protein

Servings: 4

Ingredients:

- 16 ounces uncooked tricolor spiral pasta
- ½ C. thinly sliced carrots
- 2 chopped stalks celery
- ½ C. chopped green bell pepper
- ½ C. chopped red bell pepper
- ½ C. chopped yellow bell pepper
- 1 pint halved grape tomatoes
- ½ C. chopped green onion
- 16 ounces Italian dressing
- ½ C. grated parmesan

Instructions:

1. Cook pasta according to instructions. Rinse well in cold water and place in the fridge.

2. Combine all of the chopped veggies with Italian dressing.

3. Remove cooked pasta from the fridge. Mixed chopped veggies with pasta, tossing well.

4. Transfer to serving bowl and top with parmesan cheese.

6. Red Lentil and Sweet Potato Plate

Calories 200 – 6g Fat – 5g Carb – 12g Protein

Servings: 1

Ingredients:

- 1 tbsp. olive oil
- ½ chopped onion
- 1 tsp. paprika
- 1 peeled/diced sweet potato
- 5/8 C. red lentils
- 3 sprigs of thyme
- 2 C. low-sodium vegetable stock
- 1 tsp. red wine vinegar
- Pita bread
- Choice of veggies (celery and carrot sticks, zucchini, etc.)

Instructions:

1. Combine spices together.
2. Boil red lentils according to package instructions.
3. Place sweet potato into the oven at 350 degrees for 20 minutes. Remove and let cool a bit.
4. Mix sweet potato with lentils. Then combine with spice mixture. Place in pot with veggie stock and red wine vinegar. Bring to boiling and let simmer 10 minutes till thickened.
5. Serve in a bowl alongside veggie slices and pita bread.

7. Club Salad

Calories 254 – 10g Fat – 8g Carb – 9g Protein

Servings: 2

Ingredients:

- ☒ 1 tbsp. low-fat mayo
- ☒ 2 C. chopped iceberg lettuce
- ☒ 1 slice cooked/crumbled bacon
- ☒ 1 C. grape tomatoes
- ☒ 2 slices deli turkey

Instructions:

1. Toss lettuce, bacon, tomatoes together.
2. Chop up turkey and toss with lettuce mixture.
3. Toss entire salad with mayo.

8. Sushi Sandwich

Calories 296 – 10g Fat – 5g Carb – 18g Protein

Servings: 1

Ingredients:

- 2 slices deli turkey
- ¼ C. grated mozzarella cheese
- 1 C. chopped roasted red pepper
- 1 whole wheat tortilla

Instructions:

1. Mix mozzarella and roasted red pepper together.
2. Slice pita into strips and lay out.
3. Top pita strips with deli turkey strips and mozzarella mixture.
4. Roll up tightly and enjoy your "sushi."

9. Spicy Chickpeas and Tuna

Calories 290 – 11g Fat – 4g Carb – 12g Protein

Servings: 1

Ingredients:

- ☒ 2 C. chopped romaine lettuce
- ☒ ½ C. chickpeas
- ☒ ¼ tsp. cayenne pepper
- ☒ 3 ounces light tuna in olive oil

Instructions:

1. Combine cayenne pepper and chickpeas together.
2. Combine chopped lettuce, chickpeas and tuna together.

10. Mexican Quinoa

Calories 240 – 6g Fat – 7g Carb – 11g Protein

Servings: 2

Ingredients:

- 1 diced red pepper
- Chipotle chili powder
- ¼ C. black beans
- ¼ C. corn kernels
- ½ C. cooked quinoa

Instructions:

1. Cook quinoa according to package instructions.
2. Toss quinoa with black beans, corn, and red pepper. Sprinkle with chili powder and devour.

DINNER RECIPES

1. Slow Cooker Pepperoni and Chicken

Calories 300 – 10g Fat – 4g Carb – 52g Protein

Servings: 4

Ingredients:

- ½ C. sliced black olives
- 35 halved turkey pepperonis
- ¼ tsp. red pepper flakes
- ½ tsp. basil
- 1 tsp. Italian seasoning
- 3 tbsp. tomato paste
- 1 C. low-sodium chicken broth
- 2 pounds boneless, skinless chicken breasts

Instructions:

1. Put chicken into slow cooker and season with pepper and salt.
2. Stir red pepper flakes, Italian seasoning, tomato paste, and chicken broth together and add to chicken.
3. Then add olives and pepperonis to slow cooker.
4. Cook 3 hours on high or 6 hours on low.
5. Shred chicken with tongs and mix well to soak up cooking liquids.

2. Three Cheese Penne

Calories 284 – 7g Fat – 44g Carb – 16g Protein

Servings: 8

Ingredients:

- ☒ 2 tbsp. parsley
- ☒ 1 ½ C. shredded mozzarella cheese
- ☒ ½ C. part-skim ricotta cheese
- ☒ ½ C. low-fat cottage cheese
- ☒ ¼ tsp. pepper
- ☒ ¼ tsp. salt
- ☒ ½ tsp. oregano
- ☒ ½ tsp. basil
- ☒ 1 jar pasta sauce

Instructions:

1. Heat a pot of salted water up to boiling. Cook pasta until al dente. Drain and place to the side.

2. Heat olive oil in a skillet and add garlic and onions 3 to 5 minutes till softened. Turn down heat and pour in pasta sauce. Mix in pepper, salt, oregano, and basil. Cover and cook 5 to 7 minutes.

3. Ensure oven is preheated to 350 degrees. Coat an 8x8 dish liberally.

4. Combine a cup of mozzarella, ricotta, and cottage cheese.

5. Take sauce off the heat and mix in pasta.

6. Pour half of the mixture into dish. Spread cheese mixture over the top, followed by remaining pasta and remaining cheese mixture. Sprinkle with remaining mozzarella cheese.

7. Bake 18 to 20 minutes till cheese is melted.

3. Skinny Mexican Chicken Bake

Calories 280 – 13g Fat – 15g Carb – 30g Protein

Servings: 8

Ingredients:

- ☒ 1-ounce crushed tortilla strips
- ☒ ½ C. reduced-fat shredded cheddar cheese
- ☒ 4 high fiber 9-inch tortillas
- ☒ 10-ounce can red enchilada sauce
- ☒ 2-ounces of reduced fat cream cheese
- ☒ 1 C. reduced-fat shredded Mexican cheese blend
- ☒ 1 C. chopped white onion
- ☒ 2 4-ounce cans diced green chilies
- ☒ 2 pounds boneless, skinless chicken breasts
- ☒ 2 C. reduced-sodium chicken broth

Instructions:

1. Ensure oven is preheated to 350 degrees.

2. In a skillet, combine broth and 1 can of chilies and heat to boiling. Add chicken, decrease heat and simmer 15

minutes till chicken is cooked. Make sure to turn over once during this time.

3. Take out the chicken and remove 1 cup of cooking liquid. Allow chicken to cool.

4. Shred chicken.

5. In the same skillet, heat other can of chilies and onion along with reserved cooking liquids. Sauté 3 minutes.

6. Then add cream cheese and milk, stirring till melted. Then add Mexican cheese, stirring till melted.

7. Add enchilada sauce to shredded chicken.

8. Coat a 9x13 pan and place tortillas into the pan, overlapping a bit. Top with half of the chicken mixture.

9. Repeat with other tortillas and remaining chicken mixture. Top with remaining cheddar cheese and crumbled chips.

10. With foil, cover pan and bake 15 minutes.

11. Take off foil and cook another 15 minutes.

4. Cheesy Spinach and Mushroom Lasagna Rolls

Calories 280 – 9g Fat – 23g Carb – 17g Protein

Servings: 8

Ingredients:

- ½ C. shredded mozzarella cheese
- 10-ounces chopped spinach
- 1/8 tsp. pepper
- ¼ tsp. salt
- 1 beaten egg
- ½ C. grated parmesan cheese
- 15-ounce container ricotta cheese, part-skim
- ¼ tsp. oregano
- ½ tsp. basil
- 14.5-ounce can diced tomatoes
- 23.5-ounce can pasta sauce
- 1 tbsp. minced garlic
- ½ diced onion
- 8-ounce container sliced mushrooms
- 1 tsp. extra virgin olive oil
- 8 whole wheat lasagna noodles

Instructions:

1. Ensure your oven is preheated to 350 degrees. With cooking spray, liberally coat a 7x11 dish.

2. Heat a salted pot of water up to boiling. Add lasagna noodles and cook until al dente. Drain and lay noodles out onto wax paper, covering them with a damp paper towel.

3. Warm up olive oil in a skillet and add garlic, onions, and mushrooms, cooking 3 to 4 minutes till softened.

4. Stir oregano, basil, diced tomatoes, and pasta sauce together.

5. Mix pepper, salt, egg, parmesan cheese, and ricotta cheese together. Then stir in spinach.

6. Pour half of the pasta sauce mixture into the dish.

7. Then spread about 1/3 of the cheese mixture and a tablespoon of the mushroom mixture into each of the lasagna noodles.

8. Roll filled noodles and place into the dish with the seam side down. Pour remaining pasta sauce over noodles and sprinkle with remaining mozzarella cheese.

9. With foil, cover dish and bake 30 minutes.

5. Skinny Cheeseburger Casserole

Calories 255 – 8g Fat – 21g Carb – 20g Protein

Servings: 8

Ingredients:

- 1 C. reduced-fat sharp shredded cheddar cheese
- 2 14.5-ounce cans diced tomatoes
- 1 tbsp. yellow mustard
- 2 tbsp. reduced-sugar ketchup
- 1 tbsp. Worcestershire sauce
- ¼ tsp. pepper
- ¼ salt
- ½ tsp. garlic powder
- ½ tsp. onion powder
- 1-pound lean ground beef
- 1 diced onion
- 8-ounces whole grain elbow macaroni

Instructions:

1. Ensure your oven is preheated to 350 degrees. Liberally spray a 13x9 dish with cooking spray.
2. Heat a pot of salted water to boiling and add elbow macaroni. Cook until al dente, drain and set to the side.
3. Warm up a skillet and add beef and onions, breaking up beef as it cooks for 6 to 8 minutes.
4. Add remaining ingredients to beef minus the cheese. Add macaroni, stirring well. Pour contents of skillet into the dish and cover with cheese.
5. Bake 20 to 25 minutes till cheese melts.

6. Baked Sweet and Sour Chicken

Calories 294 – 10g Fat – 25g Carb – 24g Protein

Servings: 4

Ingredients:

- 3 thinly sliced green onions
- 1 chopped yellow bell pepper
- 1 chopped red bell pepper
- 1 chopped onion
- 1/8 tsp. red pepper flakes
- 1 tsp. stevia
- 1 tsp. minced garlic
- 1 tbsp. low-sodium soy sauce
- 2 tbsp. rice vinegar
- ¼ C. reduced-sugar ketchup
- 8-ounce can pineapple chunks, packed in 100% juice
- 2 tbsp. extra virgin olive oil
- 1/3 C. + 2 tsp. cornstarch
- 1-pound boneless, skinless chicken breasts

Instructions:

1. Ensure your oven is preheated to 350 degrees. Liberally grease a 7x11 dish.

2. Cut up chicken into 1-inch cubes.

3. In a resealable bag, add 1/3 cup cornstarch and chicken. Shake bag to coat.

4. Warm up olive oil in a skillet, adding chicken in a singular layer and cooking 1 to 2 minutes till browned.

5. Drain pineapple and reserve juice.

6. Whisk remaining cornstarch, red pepper flakes, stevia, garlic, soy sauce, rice vinegar, ketchup, and reserved pineapple juice together.

7. Placed cooked chicken into the dish. Then add red and yellow bell peppers, onions, and pineapple chunks to chicken, pouring pineapple sauce mixture over veggies and chicken.

8. With foil, cover dish. Bake 45 minutes, making sure to rotate dish halfway through cooking.

9. Serve topped with green onions. Enjoy!

7. Chicken Parmesan Casserole

Calories 268 – 4g Fat – 40g Carb – 2g Protein

Servings: 8

Ingredients:

- ⅟₄ C. panko bread crumbs
- ¼ C. reduced-fat shredded parmesan cheese
- ½ C. reduced-fat shredded mozzarella cheese
- 1 tbsp. Italian seasoning
- 2 tbsp. finely chopped basil
- 3 C. low-sodium chicken broth
- 28-ounce can crushed tomatoes
- 13.5-ounce box whole wheat penne pasta
- 1-pound boneless, skinless chicken breasts

Instructions:

1. Ensure your oven is preheated to 350 degrees and liberally grease a 13x9 dish.

2. Cut up chicken into 1-inch cubes and spread into a singular layer in the bottom of the dish. Season chicken with pepper and salt and spread uncooked penne pasta over chicken.

3. Pour chicken broth and crushed tomatoes over pasta, sprinkling with Italian seasoning and basil. With foil, cover dish. Bake 45 minutes.

4. Uncover dish and top with bread crumbs and cheeses. Bake another 10 minutes to melt cheese.

8. Cheese Burrito Skillet

Calories 275 – 11g Fat – 22g Carb – 25g Protein

Servings: 6

Ingredients:

- ¾ C. 4-cheese Mexican shredded cheese
- 3 6-inch whole wheat tortillas
- 1 C. water
- 1 C. chunky salsa
- 15-ounce reduced-sodium red kidney beans
- ¼ tsp. paprika
- ½ tsp. salt
- ½ tsp. cumin
- ¼ tsp. onion powder
- ¼ tsp. garlic powder
- 1 tbsp. chili powder
- 1 pound ground turkey
- 1 diced onion
- 2 tsp. extra virgin olive oil

Optional Toppings:

- Green onions
- Yogurt
- Sour cream
- Diced tomato
- Diced avocado

Instructions:

1. Warm up olive oil in a skillet and add onion. Cook 2 to 3 minutes.

2. Add turkey to skillet, breading up as it cooks.

3. Add paprika, salt, cumin, oregano, onion powder, garlic powder, and chili powder to meat, combining well.

4. Decrease heat and add water, salsa, and beans. Simmer 4 to 5 minutes.

5. Slice tortillas into 1-inch wide strips. Add to skillet, pushing them around 2 minutes to become coated.

6. Take skillet off the heat and add cheese. Let sit 5 minutes to melt cheese.

7. Top with desired toppings before devouring.

9. Green Chili Chicken Lasagna

Calories 247 – 7g Fat – 18g Carb – 23g Protein

Servings: 9

Ingredients:

- ☒ 1 C. reduced-fat Mexican shredded cheese
- ☒ 1 C. ricotta cheese, part-skim
- ☒ 1 tsp. cumin
- ☒ 2 tbsp. chopped cilantro
- ☒ 2 4-ounce cans diced green chilies
- ☒ 10-ounce can salsa verde
- ☒ 1 C. plain Greek yogurt
- ☒ 3 C. cooked/shredded chicken
- ☒ 9 whole grain lasagna noodles

Instructions:

1. Ensure your oven is preheated to 350 degrees. Liberally spray a 13x9 dish.
2. Cook lasagna noodles along with instructions till al dente.
3. Stir a dash of pepper and salt, cumin, cilantro, green chilies, salsa verde, yogurt, and shredded chicken together.
4. Pour ¼ of the chicken mixture into bottom of the dish. Layer 3 of lasagna noodles, then 1/3 of chicken mixture, ½ cup of ricotta and ¼ cup shredded cheese.
5. Repeat layers with remaining ingredients.
6. Top with shredded cheese and bake 30 minutes.
7. Top with more cilantro and chopped tomatoes if you desire.

10. Sausage Zucchini Boats

Calories 280 – 12g Fat – 25g Carb – 22g Protein

Servings: 4

Ingredients:

- ¼ C. shredded parmesan cheese
- 1/3 C. panko bread crumbs
- 2 C. low-sugar marinara sauce
- ½ tsp. basil
- ½ tsp. cumin
- ½ tsp. pepper
- ½ tsp. salt
- ¼ tsp. red pepper flakes
- 4 diced sausage links
- 2 tbsp. minced garlic
- 1 diced yellow onion
- 1 tsp. extra virgin olive oil
- 4 zucchinis

Instructions:

1. Ensure your oven is preheated to 400 degrees. Liberally grease a 13x9 dish.

2. Cut your zucchinis in half lengthwise. Remove centers and save. Chop up centers.

3. Heat up a pot of water to boiling and add scooped out zucchini centers to pot. Cook 1 to 2 minutes. Remove and set on a plate lined with paper towels.

4. Heat up oil in a skillet and cook onions 6 to 8 minutes till they are translucent.

5. Add sausage, garlic, reserved zucchini center, basil, cumin, pepper, salt, and red pepper flakes to skillet. Cook 2 to 3 minutes, stirring well to ensure even incorporation.

6. Place ½ a cup of marinara sauce into the bottom of dish and line zucchini halves into the sauce. Fill zucchini boats with sausage mixture and pour remaining sauce over the tops.

7. Combine parmesan cheese and breadcrumbs together, then sprinkle crumbs over top of boats.

8. Spray panko crust with cooking spray.

9. Bake 20 to 25 minutes till cheese is melted and the top turns a golden brown.

DESSERT RECIPES

1. Fluff Cake

Calories 120 – 0g Fat – 0g Carb – 0g Protein

Servings: 12

Ingredients:

- ☒ 20-ounce can crush pineapple
- ☒ 16-ounce box angel food cake mix

Optional:

- ☒ Whipped topping
- ☒ Chopped fruit

Instructions:

1. Ensure your oven is preheated to 350 degrees. Grease a 13x9 pan.
2. Mix angel food cake mix with pineapple and pineapple juice. Combine well.
3. Pour batter into the pan.
4. Bake 35 to 40 minutes till golden on top.
5. Allow to cool and slice into squares. Serve with choice of fruit and whipped topping if desired.

2. Single Serving Brownie

Calories 100 – 0g Fat – 2g Carb – 1g Protein

Servings: 1

Ingredients:

- 2 tbsp. applesauce
- 1 tbsp. cocoa powder
- 1 tbsp. sweetener of choice
- 1 tbsp. flour
- Pinch of salt
- Pinch of baking soda

Instructions:

1. Combine all ingredients well.
2. Pour into a bowl and microwave 60 seconds to 90 seconds.
3. Sprinkle powdered sweetener on top if desired.

3. Skinny Oreo Cheesecake Dessert

Calories 134 – 8g Fat – 3g Carb – 0g Protein

Servings: 2 cups

Ingredients:

- 4 Oreo thins
- 1 C. fat-free cool whip
- 2 tbsp. sugar-free instant cheesecake pudding mix
- 1 C. nonfat vanilla Greek yogurt

Instructions:

1. Mix pudding mix and yogurt together till smooth. Fold in cool whip and then mix in crushed Oreo cookies.

2. Chill till you are ready to indulge!

4. Healthy Wendy's Frosty

Calories 194 – 4g Fat – 5g Carb – 0g Protein

Servings: 2

Ingredients:

- 7 ice cubes
- 2 tbsp. cool whip
- ½ tbsp. Splenda sweetener
- 1 tsp. unsweetened cocoa powder
- 1 tsp. vanilla
- 2 tbsp. sugar-free chocolate pudding mix
- 1 C. nonfat milk

Instructions:

1. Add all ingredients to a blender, pureeing till smooth and ice is chopped up. Enjoy!

5. Peach Cobbler

Calories 144 – 0.3g Fat – 32g Carb – 4g Protein

Servings: 6

Ingredients:

- 1 can of peaches in 100% juice
- 1 C. Splenda
- Dash of cinnamon
- 1 C. skim milk
- 1 C. self-rising flour

Instructions:

1. Ensure your oven is preheated to 375 degrees.
2. Mix flour, milk, and Splenda together. Then fold in peaches.
3. Grease a dish and pour in peach mixture.
4. Add cinnamon over the top.
5. Bake 30 to 35 minutes until golden in color.

6. Cherry Sorbet

Calories 142 – 0.7g Fat – 26g Carb – 10g Protein

Servings: 2

Ingredients:

- ☒ 1 tsp. sweetener
- ☒ 2 – 2 ½ tbsp. milk
- ☒ 16-ounce bag frozen, unsweetened cherries
- ☒ 5-ounce container non-fat vanilla Greek yogurt

Instructions:

1. In a blender, puree cherries and yogurt together.

2. Add sweetener and one tablespoon of milk. Blend till creamy, adding ½ a tablespoon of milk at a time till you reach a creamy and thick consistency.

7. Ingredient Healthy Indulgence Cookies

Calories 32 – 0g Fat – 5g Carb – 1g Protein

Servings: 18

Ingredients:

- 1 ¾ C. quick oats
- 2 ripe bananas

Optional Add-Ins:

- ¼ C. shredded coconut
- 1-2 tsp. vanilla
- 1/3 C. dried fruit (dates, sultanas, raisins, cranberries, etc.)
- 1/3 C. crushed nuts (walnuts, almonds, peanuts, pecans, etc.)
- ¼ C. peanut butter chips
- ¼ C. hazelnut spread
- ¼ C. cacao chips
- 1-2 tsp. honey
- ¼ C. dark chocolate chips
- 4 tbsp. peanut flour or nut butter

Instructions:

1. Ensure your oven is preheated to 350 degrees.
2. Mash your bananas and add oats, combining well.
3. Fold in any of the optional ingredients from the list.
4. With parchment paper, line a baking sheet. Drop tablespoon-sized amounts of dough onto the tray.
5. Bake 15 to 20 minutes till just golden.

8. Strawberry Oatmeal Bars

Calories 205 – 2g Fat – 4g Carb – 3g Protein

Servings: 16

Ingredients:

- ☒ 1 tbsp. sugar
- ☒ 1 tbsp. fresh lemon juice
- ☒ 2 C. diced strawberries
- ☒ 6 tbsp. melted, unsalted butter
- ☒ ¼ tsp. salt
- ☒ ¼ tsp. ginger
- ☒ 1/3 C. light brown sugar
- ☒ ¾ C. white whole wheat flour
- ☒ 1 C. old-fashioned rolled oats

Vanilla Glaze:

- ☒ 1 tbsp. milk
- ☒ ½ tsp. vanilla
- ☒ ½ C. sifted powdered sugar

Instructions:

1. Ensure your oven is preheated to 375 degrees and that a rack is placed in the center of the oven. With parchment paper, line an 8x8 dish.

2. Combine salt, ginger, brown sugar, flour, and oats together. Mix in melted butter, stirring till clumps form and all dry ingredients are moistened.

3. Reserve ½ a cup of crumble mixture and press rest into the bottom of the dish.

4. Sprinkle half the strawberries over the crumble crust in the dish, along with cornstarch.

5. Then, drizzle lemon juice and ½ a tablespoon of sugar.

6. Add remaining berries and remaining sugar. Then, sprinkle reserved crumble mixture over top of everything.

7. Bake 35 to 40 minutes till fruit becomes bubbly and crumble mixture is golden and smells toasty.

8. Prepare glaze as bars cool by whisking milk, vanilla, and sugar together till smooth.

9. Lift bars from pan, drizzle with glaze, slice and devour!

9. Mini Pineapple Upside Down Cakes

Calories 107 – 2g Fat – 20g Carb – 1g Protein

Servings: 24

Ingredients:

- 3 eggs
- 1/3 C. unsweetened applesauce
- 1 box of yellow cake mix
- 12 halved maraschino cherries
- 20-ounce can of pineapple chunks in 100% juice
- 1 C. reserved pineapple juice
- 2 tbsp. brown sugar

Instructions:

1. Ensure your oven is preheated to 350 degrees. Liberally grease a 12-count muffin tin.
2. Sprinkle ¼ tsp. of brown sugar into each muffin tin compartment.
3. Cut pineapple chunks in half and lay 2 halves into each tin, placing narrow ends together to look like a bowtie.
4. Put 1 cherry half into the center of the pineapple bowties.
5. Whisk eggs, reserved pineapple juice, applesauce, and cake mix together with a hand mixer till smooth.
6. Pour batter over filled tins.
7. Bake 12 to 15 minutes.
8. Let cool and remove by running a butter knife along the edges. Flip over, so the bottoms of the cake are the tops to reveal delicious pineapple.

10. Stuffed Baked Apples

Calories 182 – 4g Fat – 38g Carb – 5g Protein

Servings: 4

Ingredients:

- ¼ tsp. vanilla
- 1 tsp. orange zest
- 2 tbsp. cream cheese
- 1 tsp. cinnamon
- 2 tbsp. brown sugar
- ¼ C. instant oats
- 4 apples

Instructions:

1. Ensure your oven is preheated to 375 degrees.
2. Remove cores from apples, making sure you don't cut through them.
3. Combine cinnamon, brown sugar, and oats.
4. Mix vanilla, orange zest, and cream cheese together.
5. Spoon a tablespoon of cream cheese mixture into each apple and fill the rest of apples with oat mixture.
6. Place filled applies to a baking dish. Pour water around apple just enough to cover the bottom about 1 centimeter.
7. With foil, loosely cover pan. Bake 20 minutes.
8. Uncover dish and bake another 25 to 30 minutes.

Conclusion

I want to congratulate you for making it to the end of *The Complete Low-Calorie Cookbook*!

I hope that you found this book to be a great guide as you make the plunge in really digging deep to change your overall lifestyle for the better. This books not only holds a nice variety of meals for all portions of the day but if used with other healthy habits, you are the one that holds the power over your health. It's time to stop letting convenient, fast food and junk foods rule your life.

If you are ready to stop feeling crummy about your self-image and want to feel better physically, then it's now up to you to take the reins of your life and get that control back!

I am sure you found a number of recipes in this book that caught your eye and made your mouth water; start with those recipes first! Then, make your way through the remaining recipes. I have no doubt that you will begin to notice a difference in your overall energy and health as you fuel your body with delicious, healthy, low-carb meals and treats!

I hope that with this book, you are able to achieve your health and fitness goals, whatever they may be.

Finally, if you found this book useful in anyway, a review on Amazon is always appreciated!

CPSIA information can be obtained
at www.ICGtesting.com
Printed in the USA
LVHW080049230421
685200LV00045B/36

9 781913 796907